DIETS OF THE WORLD

18 DIETS EXPLAINED

MUJJA SAIKUMAR

ISBN 979-888546390-4

Dedicated to YOU and to all my supporters and well wishers.

#healthyindia

Contents

Introduction *vii*

Diets Of The World

1. Paleo Diet 3
2. Atkins Diet 5
3. Ketogenic Diet 7
4. Mediterranean Diet 9
5. The Nordic Diet 11
6. Standard American Diet 12
7. Indian Diet 13
8. Raw Food Diet 14
9. Vegetarian Diet 15
10. Vegan Diet 16
11. The Dukan Diet 18
12. The Zone Diet 20
13. Weight Watchers Diet 21
14. Hcg Diet 23
15. Blood Type Diet 25
16. Gm Diet 26
17. South Beach Diet 28
18. Intermittent Fasting 30

Final Word 33

Introduction

You only live once, for a short period of time. So live well.

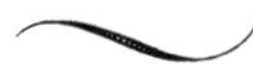

I still remember the day when I thought it is necessary to write this book. Most of the questions on my Instagram Dm's and polls are about the type of diet they should follow for a particular health goal. Though I write a lot on such health and fitness topics on my blog - www.themusclyadvisor.com, I thought it is better to mention the most common diet types you might hear in one place.

So, What is a Diet?

In short, it is the practice of eating food in a regular intervals to decrease, maintain, or increase body weight, or to prevent diseases and to maintain health. Diet can also refer to the food and drink a person consumes daily and the mental and physical circumstances connected to eating. Nutrition and diet is directly proportional to your Health. If the word "Diet" immediately make you think of weight-loss or weight-gain regimen, you are probably not alone. Many people often ask or google the same. To answer this questions you need to know the most common diets available in the world. That is where this book stands for.

A total of 18 diet types are mentioned in this book. This book does not deal with the advantages and disadvantages of a diet type. The sole aim of this Book is to provide a basic overview on 18 of the most common and well known diets around the globe. Remember, this book is not a recommendation for you to follow a particular type of diet.

Much love,
Mujja Saikumar
(Author)

Diets of the World

CHAPTER ONE

PALEO DIET

There is a reason for mentioning this diet in the first place. Paleo diet is otherwise called as Paleolithic diet, Stone Age diet, hunter-gatherer diet and caveman diet. As the name suggests, this diet mimics the hunters and gatherers. This type of diet does not contain any of the processed or unnatural foods. It is the natural way of eating from our ancestors before agriculture developed.

Paleo diet restricts sugar intake in all artificial and processed forms and the only sugars in the paleo diet comes from fruits. Anything that available in the nature is taken as it is like a caveman, focusing only on lean meat, fish, seeds, fruits and vegetables. This diet is basically a low-carb diet. It may be a very restrictive type of diet to now-a-days people. The theory of paleo diet is that modern diseases are linked to modern diets. Several studies are there to prove the benefits of paleo diet. Paleo diet helps in weight loss. In 2008, a study conducted by European Journal of Clinical Nutrition on 14 healthy volunteers for 3 weeks to study effects of short-term intervention with a paleolithic diet. This study claims that the participants lost an average of 5 pounds, and waist circumference decreased by 0.7 inches.

This diet is helpful for people with type-2 Diabetes. In 2009, a study conducted on 13 individuals with type-2 diabetes by a medical journal, cardiovascular diabetology. This study states that blood sugar levels decreased by 0.4% and HDL(High Density Lipoprotein) cholesterol rose by 3 mg/dL than the people who follow typical diabetes diet. Some researches claims several health benefits of a Paleolithic diet. A Paleolithic diet reduces inflammation and digestive stress, Increased and more stable energy levels, Less or no bloating, decreased gas and Sustained weight loss. These studies are too small with the number of participants ranging from 9–29 and too short in duration to form a definitive conclusion about the paleo diet.

However, the diet is growing in popularity in recent years. and research on its effectiveness continues and therefore, more evidence may emerge to support the health benefits of the paleo diet.

What to eat in Paleo Diet:

In paleo diet, You are allowed to eat meats from grass fed animals like beef, chicken, pork, fish, turkey, Pasture-raised Eggs, Non-starchy Vegetables like broccoli, cauliflower, Tomato etc..All type of Fruits, Seeds, Olive oil, coconut oil, Salt, Ginger, natural honey and all other 100% naturally occurring foods.

What to avoid in Paleo Diet:

Foods like grains, rice, barley, oats, cereals, potatoes, legumes, sugars, candy, doughnuts, softdrinks, oats, vegetable oils, farm animals, even dairy products like yogurt, milk, ghee, icecream, curd and any processed foods or simply anything that comes in wrapper are restricted.

CHAPTER TWO

Atkins Diet

The Atkins diet is devised by the physician Dr. Robert C. Atkins, in 1972. It is considered to be a low-carb diet, usually claims that you can lose weight while eating as much protein and fat without counting calories, as long as you avoid foods high in carbs. In the past decade, over 15 studies have shown that low-carb diets are effective for weight loss and can lead to various health benefits. This diet is considered among the fad diets and unhealthy because of it's high saturated fat content. However, new studies proved that saturated fat is harmless and helps in raising HDL - High Density Lipoprotein(good cholesterol). Researches have also shown that Saturated fats does not raise LDL - Low Density Lipoprotein (bad cholesterol).

Depending on your goal Atkins Diet has four phases.

Phase 1: This is a introduction phase. In this phase you should eat only 20 grams or less carbohydrates in a day for two week including high-protein and high-fat. This phase kick starts the weight loss.

Phase 2: This is a balancing phase. In this phase you should add more nuts, low-carb vegetables and some amount of fruits. You should stay in this phase until you're about 4.5 kilograms from your goal weight.

Phase 3: This is a pre-maintenance or fine- tuning phase. When you are close to your goal weight you should add more carbs untill your weightloss slows down.

Phase 4: This is a lifetime maintenance phase. Here you can eat more healthy carbs as your body can tolerate without regaining weight, and then you continue this way of eating. What to eat: Low carb foods, lean protein, and healthy fats

What to eat in Atkins Diet:

Lean meats like Beef, pork, lamb, chicken and others.
Fatty fishes and seafoods like Salmon, trout, sardines, etc.
Eggs: The healthiest eggs are omega-3 enriched or pastured.
Low-carb vegetables: Kale, spinach, broccoli, asparagus and others.
Full-fat dairy like butter, cheese, cream, yogurt.
Nuts and seeds and Healthy fats like extra virgin olive oil, coconut oil, avocados and avocado oil.

What to avoid in Atkins Diet:

Sugary foods like soft drinks, icecream, fruit juices, cakes, chocolates.
Grains like wheat, rice, barley.
Vegetable oils or the hydrogenated oils like soyoil, corn oil etc..
High carb fruits like Apples, bananas, grapes.
Legumes and the starchy foods like potato, sweet potato.

CHAPTER THREE

KETOGENIC DIET

Ketogenic diet Or simply keto diet. Keto diet is referred to a low carb, high fat diet. This diet got more popularity in the recent times. The idea of keto diet is to get more calories from proteins and fats and less from carbohydrates. Easily digesting carbs(simple carbs), refined carbs should be restricted. If you eat less carbs your body eventually runs out of fuel and then you'll start to break down protein and fat for energy, eventually aids in weight loss. And this metabolic state called ketosis. This diet is mainly focused on weight loss rather than the persuit of health benefits. Infact, over 18 studies show that this type of diet can support weight loss and improve your health.

Keto diets may even have benefits against diabetes, cancer, epilepsy and Alzheimer's disease and some other studies have shown that decreasing simple, refined and processed carb intake, a ketogenic diet could reduce acne symptoms, reduce risk of certain cancers like breast and colon cancer, improve heart health, reduces seizures and also Improves PCOS symptoms in women. Mostly, endurance athletes prefer keto diet because it helps to keep muscle-to-fat ratio and raises the amount of oxygen that body is able to use. It is better to consult your doctor first to find out if it's safe for you to try a ketogenic diet, especially if you have type 1 diabetes.

There are several versions of the ketogenic diet, namely:

Standard ketogenic diet (SKD): This is a very low-carb, moderate-protein and high-fat diet. i.e., 75% fats, 20% protein and 5% carbs of the total calorie intake. For instance, if you are following a 2,000 calorie diet. Then, 75% of calories, that means 1500 calories should come from fats, and 20% calories, that is 400 calories from protein, and the remaining 100 calories from carbs.

Cyclical ketogenic diet (CKD): This diet involves eating high carb diets periodically, such as 5 ketogenic days followed by 2 high-carb days.

Targeted ketogenic diet (TKD): This diet allows you to add carbs around workouts.

High-protein ketogenic diet(HKD): This type is same as standard ketogenic diet, but includes more protein. i.e., 60% fat, 35% protein and 5% carbs of the total calorie intake.

What to eat in Ketogenic Diet:

Sea foods, Low-Carb Vegetables, Cheese, Avocados, Meat and Poultry, Eggs, Coconut oil, Olive oil, Nuts and seeds, Plain Greek Yogurt and Cottage Cheese, Berries, Butter and Cream, Unsweetened Coffee and Tea, Dark Chocolate and Cocoa Powder.

What to avoid in Ketogenic Diet:

All fruits, Grains like rice, barley, oats, starches, legumes, sugar, sweet treats, alcohol, condiments like ketchup, BBQ sauce.. and Low-fat dairy.

CHAPTER FOUR

Mediterranean Diet

Mediterranean diet is inspired by the healthy traditional flavours and cooking methods of the countries around Mediterranean sea, such as Greece, Croatia, France, Spain and Italy. It is a natural way of eating. Interest in the Mediterranean diet began back in the 1950's and 1960's. The Mediterranean diet blends the basics of heart healthy eating. The Mediterranean diet has no one right way to follow as it varies by country and region.

The reason why people love the Mediterranean diet is that, it allows of moderate amounts of red wine. That is approximately, 5 ounces (oz) or less each day for women (one glass) and no more than 10 oz daily for men (two glasses). This diet is quite popular because it isn't restrictive and have more health benefits. People in the countries around Mediterranean sea are known for having some of the lowest rates of heart disease, diabetes, metabolic syndrome and cancer worldwide. There are studies to claim the health benefits of Mediterranean diet. The PERDIMED study on 7,447 individuals with a high risk of heart disease and the participants made follow one of these diets for almost 5 years.

1. Mediterranean diet with added extra virgin olive oil
2. Mediterranean diet with added nuts.

This study states that the risk of combined heart attack, stroke, and death from heart disease was lower by 31% in the people who follow Mediterranean + Olive Oil and 28% in the people who follow Mediterranean + Nuts and it is also found that a Mediterranean diet supplemented with nuts may help reverse metabolic syndrome.

What to eat in Mediterranean Diet:

Fish, and other seafoods, is a staple in the Mediterranean diet.
The Mediterranean diet is mostly plant based.
Eating plenty of starchy foods, such as bread and pasta
Eating plenty of fruit, vegetables, herbs, nuts, beans and whole grains.
Plant oils like extra-virgin olive oil.
Moderate amounts of dairy, poultry and eggs are also central to the Mediterranean Diet.
Red wine, Red meat(ocassionally).

What to avoid in Mediterranean Diet:

Sugars like Candy, Donuts, Pastries, Soft Drinks, Table Sugar, Ice-creams, Refined Grains, Diary, Factory animals, Vegetable Oils, Trans fats or simply Any Processed Foods or Anything that comes in a wrapper.

CHAPTER FIVE

The Nordic Diet

In 2004, this diet is created by a group of nutritionists. The "Nordic diet" is not really about weight loss. It is based on their traditional ways of eating. This diet incorporates foods commonly eaten by people in the Nordic countries like Denmark, Iceland, Norway, Finland, and Sweden. This diet emphasizes whole grains such as barley, rye and oats, berries, vegetables, fatty fish and legumes, and it is low in sweets and red meat. It's quite similar to the Mediterranean diet.

Both Mediterranean diet and Nordic diets are rich in plant based foods but instead of olive oil, the Nordic diet is rich in rapeseed oil or otherwise known as canola oil. There are several health benefitss of consuming plant based foods. The Nordic diet reduces diastolic blood pressure. However, The Nordic diet is not very effective at lowering blood sugar levels.

What to eat in Nordic Diet:

Mostly Cook at home, Fruits, Less processed, less sugary foods, berries, vegetables, legumes, potatoes, whole grains, nuts, seeds, rye breads, fish, seafood, low-fat dairy, herbs, spices, and rapeseed (canola) oil, game meats, free-range eggs, cheese, and yogurt, other red meats (rarely).

What to avoid in Nordic Diet:

Soft drinks, added sugars, processed meats, food additives, olive oil and refined fast foods

CHAPTER SIX

Standard American Diet

Standard American diet or simply SAD diet can also be called as Western pattern diet (WPD). More than 60% of the calories that Americans eat are from processed foods. This diet mostly contains preservatives, added sugars and other unnatural substances.

Excess consumption of unnatural foods are the primary cause of obesity and diabetes and other related diseases. Studies have proved that the SAD for a short period of time is ok but if taken for a long, this diet may result in several health issues. It is no wonder that Americans are deficit in fiber. This type of diet increases body weight and that is the reason why 70 million adults in U.S. are obese and 99 million are overweight. Being overweight or obese increase the risk of several diseases such as Diabetes, High blood pressure, inflammation, Heart Stroke, Osteoarthritis and GERD.

Standard American diet looks like:

Red meat, processed meat, packaged foods, candy and sweets, fried foods, conventionally-raised animal products, refined grains, potatoes, high-fructose corn syrup and high-sugar drinks.

What to eat to be healthy:

Fruits, vegetables, whole grains, grass-fed animal products, low fat dairy, fish, nuts, and seeds and other natural foods.

CHAPTER SEVEN

Indian Diet

Indian cuisine is known for its spices, fresh herbs and wide variety of flavors. Indian diet is generally a high carb based diet. Indian diet has a wide variety options to opt. It has many cuisines like south Indian diet, Gujarati diet, North Indian diet and so forth. Diet varies a lot in every state in India. Though diets vary throughout India, most people follow plant-based diet. Around 80-85% of the Indian population practices a vegetarian diet. The Indian diets emphasizes a high intake of vegetables, lentils and fruits, as well as a low consumption of meat. Indian diets are nutritious, filling and very tasty. Plant-based diets have been associated with many health benefits, including a lower risk of heart disease and encourage weight loss.

Macro split of typical Indian diet: (% of the total calorie intake)

P-25 F-25 C-50

P-25 F-35 C-40

P-30 F-40 C-30

Where P,F and C are protein, fats and carbs respectively.

What to eat in an Indian Diet:

All the foods that are available in India like Vegetables, Fruits, Nuts and Seeds, Legumes, Roots and tubers, Whole grains, full fat dairy, olive oil, avacado, tofu, paneer, lentils, eggs, chicken, meat and so forth.

What to avoid in an Indian Diet:

Sugars, Refined grains, High fat foods, Trans fats, Refined oils, Refined grains like white pasta, white bread and sweeteners like honey, jaggery and all Processed foods.

CHAPTER EIGHT

Raw Food Diet

It is otherwise called as Raw foodism or Rawism. As the name suggests, the person should eat uncooked and unprocessed food, preferably organic and drinks that are truly plant based. Raw food diets may include a selection of fruits, vegetables, nuts, seeds, and dairy products but generally not foods that have been pasteurized, homogenized, or produced with the use of food additives.

Weight loss is not the main aim of raw foods, but switching to raw foods may lead to weight loss sometimes. Raw foods are rich in fiber, vitamins and minerals. There are some studies that claim, cooking destroys water soluble vitamins i.e., vitamin B and vitamin C. By eliminating processed and pasteurized foods, it is less likely to cause cardiovascular diseases. Some people consider eating raw chicken, meat and eggs. According to the Centers for Disease Control (CDC), uncooked animal products are most likely to cause food poisoning.

What to eat in Raw Food Diet:

Raw fruits and raw vegetables, dried fruits and vegetables, soaked and sprouted beans, other legumes, grains, raw nuts and seeds, nut milks, including almond milk, coconut milk, olive oil or coconut oil, dried fruits.

What to avoid in Raw Food Diet:

All cooked or processed foods, refined oils, table salt, refined sugars and flour, coffee, tea, and alcohol, pasta.

CHAPTER NINE

Vegetarian Diet

Vegetarian diet involves plant foods, some animal products honey, milk, ghee, and eggs. And involves abstaining from eating meat, fish and poultry. some studies estimate that over 18% of the Global population are vegetarians. The reason why most people opt vegetarian diet is because of its health benefits, or religious, or personal reasons. studies show that a meat-free diet can lead to better health for several reasons. Vegetarians have better diet quality that the diet includes meat. There are several variations of vegetarian diets are there.

Lacto-ovo-vegetarian diet: The word lacto is related to milk and the word ovo is related to eggs. As the name suggests, this diet eliminates meat, fish and poultry but allows eggs and dairy products.

Lacto-vegetarian diet: As the name suggests, this diet eliminates meat, fish, poultry and eggs but allows dairy products.

Ovo-vegetarian diet: This diet eliminates meat, fish, poultry and dairy products but allows eggs.

Pescetarian diet: This variation eliminates meat and poultry but allows fish and it allows eggs and dairy products occassionally.

Vegan diet: This diet is quite popular. This diet 100% plant based and 0% animal based. It eliminates meat, fish, poultry, eggs and dairy products, even honey - as it made by honey bees.

Flexitarian diet: A mostly vegetarian diet that comes with occasional meat, fish or poultry.

CHAPTER TEN

VEGAN DIET

A vegan diet is a type of vegetarian diet, as mentioned in the previous chapter. It is the most popular diet among the vegetarian diet types. A vegan diet is exclusively based on plant foods. They are rich in fiber. A vegan diet excludes all animal products in all forms. Even honey is eliminated as it is made by Honey bees. There are several ways to follow a vegan diet like Whole-food vegan diet, Raw-food vegan diet, The starch solution, 80/10/10 so on and so forth, but scientific research rarely differentiates between the different types.

The vegan diet became very popular this days. Some vegans do it to improve their health and Others stay away from meat because they don't want to harm animals or because they want to protect the environment or to maintain ecological balance. Going vegan is the best way to cut down daily calories. It has several health benefits. Some researches have proved that Vegans are also less likely to get diabetes and some kinds of cancer. In some cases, it may also increase the risk of nutrient deficiencies.

Avoiding animal based foods can shortchange you on a few nutrients, like protein, calcium, omega-3 fatty acids, zinc, and vitamin B12. Protein is required for all muscle tissues and to power all the chemical reactions in your body. Calcium strengthens your bones and teeth. Omega-3 fatty acids protects your heart and brain. These nutrients are especially important for childs growth and for pregnant women. However, there are substituents available for most of these essential nutrients in plant-based foods.

What to eat in Vegan Diet:

All plant based foods like vegetables, fruits, nuts, seeds, legumes, lentils, wheat, barley, coconut oil, avocado oil, tubers and yams, dairy alternatives like soy milk, coconut milk etc....

What to avoid in Vegan Diet:

All animal based foods such as Eggs, milk, meat, honey, dairy and dairy products.

CHAPTER ELEVEN

THE DUKAN DIET

In 1975, Pierre Dukan, a former nutritionist, developed a diet and named after him, The Dukan diet. The Dukan diet is a high protein, low carbohydrate eating plan especially designed for weight loss in obese people. The Dukan Diet claims to produce permanent weight loss without hunger. The dukan diet focuses on natural foods rather than packed foods. On this dukan diet only 100 foods are allowed. Out of which 68 are protein foods and 32 are vegetables. This diet is not calorie restricted. It is fine to eat anything as long as you are in those list of 100 foods provided. Increasing protein intake helps you in weight loss and gain muscle. The dukan diet can be explained in four phases.

Phase 1: The attack phase First 10 days, the dieter can eat unlimited lean protein including 1.5 tablespoon of oat bran and at least 6-8 cups of water per day. Increase more lean protein is more likely to kick-start the metabolism.

Phase 2: The cruise phase In this phase the dieter is asked to eat Non-starchy Vegetables in the alternate days plus 2 tablespoons of oat bran every day. Usually this phase continues several months or even a year.

Phase 3: The consolidation phase This diet continues 5 days for every pound lost in phases 1 and 2. This stage does not aim to lose weight, but to avoid regaining it. You can have unlimited servings of lean protein and veggies plus 2.5 tablespoons of oat bran daily.

Phase 4: Stabilization Phase In this phase the dieter can eat whatever they want in those 100 foods. However, they can have one full protein day in a week and 3 tbsp of oat bran each day. Atleast 30 minutes of exercise is recommended. If a person gains weight again, he/she should go with phase 2 or 3.

What to eat in Dukan Diet:

The list of 100 foods is provided in their official website.

CHAPTER TWELVE

THE ZONE DIET

The Zone diet was created by Barry Sears, a biochemist. Sears believes diet-induced inflammation, is the reason we gain weight, grow sick, and age faster. The idea behind the Zone diet is that those who follow it will reset their metabolism, diabetes, and other chronic health conditions. Carbs, protein, and fat are all allowed on the zone diet, but in a specific ratios. It aims for a nutritional balance of 30% protein, 30% fats and 40% carbs preferably low GI(glycemic index) foods in all meals and snacks.

Low GI foods take more time to digest and are less likely to cause a blood sugar spike after eating. The diet advocates eating five times a day with 3 meals and 2 snacks. It encourages people to consume healthy fats and antioxidants, including omega-3 fats. There are several Benefits of being in the Zone. Losing excess body fat, Maintaining wellness, it may also help you to think better.

What to eat in the Zone Diet:

Healthy carbs that are low on the glycemic index (simply complex carbs), egg whites, fish, poultry, lean beef or low-fat dairy, mono-unsaturated fats include olive oil, avocado, or almonds.

What to avoid in the Zone Diet:

Starchy vegetables, carbs that are high on tge glycemic index (simple carbs), Transfats, softdrinks, alcohol.

CHAPTER THIRTEEN

WEIGHT WATCHERS DIET

Weight watchers diet, popularly known as WW diet is a commercial diet founded by Jean Nidetch in 1963 out of her Queens, New York home. She created a network of weight watchers. Now, Weight Watchers may be a huge company, with branches everywhere in the world. Dieters will join either physically and attend regular conferences, or online. The Weight Watchers diet is aiming to achieve a weight loss of 0.5 to 1.0 kg per week, which is the medically accepted standard rate of a viable weight loss strategy. This diet doesn't involve on calculating the calories. It is based on a "smart points" system. Weight Watchers comes up with your plan by having you answer a series of questions about yourself, including your eating and activity habits. Then it gives you your own daily budget of points for food and motivates you to not exceed it.

In Weight watchers diet every food in their list has a point value. Assume it like 10, 20, 18, 9...... For instance, if weight watchers give you 100 points limit, then you should eat within the point limit throughout the day.

Only fruits and non-starchy vegetables were rated zero points. The foods which are high in protein is considered to have minimum point value and the goods which are high in sugars is considered to have high point value. If you observe this, the weight watchers diet has very less or no restriction in eating vegetables and protein rich foods, just as other healthy diets but in an interesting and exciting approach.

The dieters can make healthier choices depending on the suggested smart points, rather than calories. Usually this smart points suggestion will be low for dieters whose goal is weight loss and more for dieters whose goal is weight gain.

What to eat Weight Watchers Diet:

There is no food restriction in this diet.

CHAPTER FOURTEEN

HCG DIET

HCG - Human Chorionic Gonadotropin. The HCG diet is an extreme weight loss diet claiming to lose 0.5 - 1 kg per day. It is an ultra-low-calorie diet of 500 calories per day along with HCG supplement ingestion as drops or injections. The HCG diet is has been discredited by scientists and listed on the top of fad diets that promises magical results with a lot of health benefits. The Food and Drug Administration (FDA) call this diet illegal and dangerous.

Human Chorionic Gonadotropin is a hormone present at high levels in early pregnancy and also used to treat fertility issues in both men and women. Some researches claims that the use of HCG increase certain cancer risks. However, an ultra-low-calorie diet alone is likely to cause weight loss. This is proved through a study that conducted on two different group of people. One group of people is provided with ultra low calorie diet with HCG supplement and the other group is provided with the same ultra low calorie diet and placebo injection. The results were found to be identical. This diet aims for overall weight loss rather that fatloss.

This diet involves in three phases.

Phase 1: It is a loading phase where you start taking HCG supplement and high calorie foods for the first 2 days.

Phase 2: It is weightloss phase where you eat an ultre low calorie diet of 500 calories along with HCG supplement. This phase continues upto 8 weeks.

Phase 3: It is a maintenance phase where you stop taking HCG supplements and increase calorie intake gradually.

What to eat in HCG Diet:

Some fruits, non starchy vegetables, lean meat.

What to avoid in HCG Diet:

Fatty foods, starchy vegetables, added sugar, soft drinks, dairy, and other processed foods that are rich in calories.

CHAPTER FIFTEEN

Blood Type Diet

The blood type diet is popularized by Dr. Peter D'Adamo, a naturopathic physician, in 1996. This diet lacks significant evidence to support its claims of effectiveness. The scope of Blood Type Diet is to limit lectins, proteins that bind to sugar molecules, based on your blood type. These diets are based on the ABO blood group system. This is derived from the idea that lectins can negatively impact some blood types more than others.

Group O is considered as the ancestral blood group in humans so their diet should resemble hunter-gatherer era. Those with type O blood should choose animal protein foods like meat, fish, poultry, dairy, eggs, fresh vegetables and fruit but limit grains, beans, and legumes.

Group A is considered as the cultivator and their diet should resemble the early agriculture era. Those with type A blood should choose vegetarian diet, diet rich in plants, seafoods, turkey but avoid meat.

Group B was believed to originate in nomadic tribes. Those with type B blood are considered to benefit from consumption of dairy products, meat, fruit, dairy, seafood, and grains. However, they should avoid wheat, corn, lentils, tomatoes and a few other foods.

Group AB is described as a mix between groups A and B. They should avoid wheat, corn, lentils, kidney beans, beef and chicken.

In 2013, a study conducted by The American Society of Clinical Nutrition on the Blood Type Diet and concluded that there was no evidence found to claim the benefits associated with the Blood Type Diet. However, research indicates that lectins(proteins that bind to carbohydrates) have similar effects on all blood types and do not impact one blood type over another. This is considered as the fad diets among several authors. However, one thing is clear that consuming more lean protein, fruits, and vegetables has benefits.

CHAPTER SIXTEEN

GM DIET

The GM diet is also known as General Motor diet. The GM diet was created for the employees of General Motors in 1985 to help their employees to deal with their weight issues. It is a seven day diet, each with a strict rules. This diet promises to lose 14-15 pounds of weight in just a week. This diet may be repeated for a multiple times to to achieve your long-term weight goals recommend with a gap of 5-7 days. There is no restrictions on the quantity of the food and there is a restriction on the type of food you eat. Table sugar, processed foods, and alcohol is completely eliminated.

The GM diet involves in weight loss including muscle loss which is not actually good. However, GM diet is your temporary solution for weight loss. It is considered to be the worst diet in the health prospective. The fixed seven day pattern of the GM diet looks like,

Day 1 Include all types of fruits except banana. No salt, no added sugars. In the first day itself the person feels weight changes.

Day 2 Include only Vegetables either cooked or raw without oil. No restriction on the quantity.

Day 3 Include a combination of fruits and vegetables avoiding banana and potato. Quantity is not restricted.

Day 4 Consume only bananas and milk.

Day 5 Consume Brown rice, Tomatoes and lean protein. Like chicken, fish and in some cases lean paneer.

Day 6 Consume Brown rice, vegetables and lean protein. Avoid potato, legumes and beans as they are high in calories.

Day 7 Take Brown rice, Vegetables, lean protein and fruits or fruit juices.

What to eat in GM Diet:

There is no pretty much restriction on food.

What to avoid in GM Diet:

Added sugars, table salt, processed foods, alcohol, fried foods and trans fats.

CHAPTER SEVENTEEN

South Beach Diet

The South Beach Diet, otherwise called as modified low-carbohydrate diet is developed by Dr.Arthur Agatston. This is not a traditional low-carb diet but it focuses on good carbs and good fats. Mostly, the foods with low Glycemic index value is preferred because these foods digest more slowly than the other and they release energy over time. This helps people to feel full for a longer period of time and prevent spikes in blood sugar level.

Firstly, this diet is aimed to lower the risk of heart disease, but it rapidly became popular for losing weight. This diet involves in 3 stages.

Stage 1 aims for rapid weight loss i.e., approx. 15lbs in the first two weeks. This stage aims to eliminate cravings and stabilizing blood-sugar levels.

In **stage 2**, Some healthy carbs such as whole-wheat breads, whole-wheat pasta, brown rice, fruits and more vegetables low on GI are added in this stage. This stage continues till you reach your goal weight.

Stage 3 is a maintaining phase. It is about maintaining an ideal body weight over a long period of time. You can go back to stage 1 or 2, if the food cravings return, or if weight increases.

What to eat in the South Beach Diet:

Lean meats, chicken, turkey, fish, tofu, eggs, low fat cheese, nuts, beans, non starchy vegetables, low-fat dairy, olive oil, coconut oil and some other healthy carbs and fats.

What to avoid in the South Beach Diet:

Bread, rice, potatoes, pasta, fruits, alcohol, soft drinks, sugary foods such as cake, cookies, candy and ice cream.

CHAPTER EIGHTEEN

INTERMITTENT FASTING

Intermittent fasting, also known as intermittent energy restriction, is a voluntary fasting over a period of time and having meals in a given non-fasting period. Intermittent fasting is a health trend in recent years. Many studies shows that this can cause weight loss, improve metabolic health, reduce the risk of diet related diseases. The American Heart Association (AHA) states that intermittent fasting may help in weight loss, reduce insulin resistance, and lower the risk of cardio-metabolic diseases.

A study in 2019 concluded that intermittent fasting may help with obesity, insulin resistance, dyslipidemia(abnormal amount of lipids in the blood), hypertension, and inflammation. There are three main methods to do intermittent fasting. They are alternate-day fasting, periodic fasting, and time-restricted feeding.

Alternate-day fasting: It involves fasting for 24 hours in alternate days and eating 25-30% less than the daily energy required in non-fasting days.

Periodic fasting: It is also called as 5:2 diet or simply Eat-stop-eat method. The periodic fasting involves eating normally 5 days a day and 2 whole days fasting in the alternate days or calories are restricted to 500 calories for women and 600 calories for men on this fasting days.

Time-restricted feeding: This is the quite popular intermittent fasting method. It involves eating only during a certain number of hours in a day. This type of intermittent fasting has several variations like 16:8, 12:12, 18:6.

16:8 type involves fasting for 16 hours a day and 8 hours of feeding time. In the same way, 12:12 is 12 hours of fasting followed by 12 hours of feeding time and similarly, 18:6.

What to eat in Intermittent Fasting:

Intermittent fasting is a time restricted method to reduce calorie intake. Generally, you can have normal healthy foods.

What to avoid in Intermittent Fasting:

High fat foods, sugars, coke, soft drinks, alcohol and All Processed foods.

Final Word

Now, you probably be thinking of the best diet among those mentioned in this book. Let me make it clear for you.

Whether it is weight loss or weight gain, a balanced diet plays a vital role. Opting for a balanced, and varied diet with an adequate amount of macros and micros is an important step towards a healthy lifestyle. Now, if you observe all the diets mentioned in this book, you can see that all the diet types suggest you to avoid alcohol, foods that are rich in sugar. Healthy eating can also prevent several health complications such as obesity, cardiovascular diseases, diabetes and improves energy, allows you to sleep better, and improve brain function. There is no best diet in the world. The one that suits you and gives results is the best one for you. However, *along with a balanced diet, fitness is important.*

Thank you so much for reading Diets of the World - A basic introduction. There's no shortage of Nutrition, Diet and Fitness books out there, so I'm grateful that you've chosen to read mine. That means a lot to me.

ABOUT ME

I'm Mujja Saikumar. I live in Andhrapradesh, India. I love learning new skills. I'm an Aeronautical Engineering graduate and a Fitness blogger(https://www.themusclyadvisor.com/). I also had an Internationally accredited diploma in Fitness, Nutrition and Diet planning.

I hope you enjoy my book content as much as I enjoy offering them to you. If you have any questions or comments, please don't hesitate to contact me. We're dedicated to giving you the very best health and fitness content.

Read our Blogs - **www.themusclyadvisor.com**

Our Social Media - **The Muscly Advisor.**

9 798885 463904

Printed by Libri Plureos GmbH in Hamburg,
Germany